Ageless Vitality

The Complete Guide to Intermittent Fasting for Women Over 50

By
Aubrey Wheatly

Table of Contents

Introduction

Hello and welcome to "Ageless Vitality: The Ultimate Guide to Intermittent Fasting for Women Over 50." In the pages that follow, we set out on a transforming journey that aims to reveal the keys to women's health and vitality in their later years.

Our bodies experience some astonishing changes as we become older, both in terms of physiology and way of life. It's critical to modify our health and wellness policies in light of the specific possibilities and problems that these changes often bring. For women over 50 who want to have the healthiest, most fulfilling lives possible, intermittent fasting, a tried-and-true and scientifically supported approach to nutrition, has emerged as a potent weapon.

This manual has been particularly designed with the needs and goals of women in this age range in mind. If you're new to intermittent fasting or you've tried it before, you'll discover a lot of knowledge, useful tips, and motivational tales on these pages.

So, whether you want to lose excess weight, get more energy, balance your hormones, or just set off on a trip to ageless vitality, this book is your dependable travel partner. It's time to realize intermittent fasting's enormous potential and start along the road to a healthier, happier, and more fulfilling existence.

Do you have the courage to embrace "Ageless Vitality"? Join me as we set off on this fascinating excursion.

Why Intermittent Fasting Matters for Women Over 50

It's advisable to consider intermittent fasting as a way to improve your health and energy for the following reasons:

Intermittent fasting may help slow down the aging process, lower the risk of illnesses associated with aging, and increase lifespan.

- Hormonal Harmony: Women over 50 often undergo hormonal changes. Particularly during menopause, intermittent fasting may be quite beneficial for maintaining hormone balance.
- Weight management: As people age, it is harder to maintain a healthy weight. An efficient and long-lasting method of controlling weight and body composition is intermittent fasting.
- Increased Energy: Managing your dietary habits may increase your energy levels, mental clarity, and general vigor.
- Intermittent fasting may lower the chance of developing some chronic illnesses, including diabetes, heart disease, and

certain kinds of cancer, according to research.

- Intermittent fasting gives you the ability to regulate your diet and well-being, giving you a feeling of confidence and success.

What to Expect from This Guide

In "Ageless Vitality: The Ultimate Guide to Intermittent Fasting for Women Over 50," we've created a thorough guide aimed at giving you the information, resources, and motivation needed to fully realize the transforming power of intermittent fasting. What to anticipate from this guide is as follows:

- **Detailed Comprehension:** Initially, we'll build the groundwork by giving you a thorough grasp of what intermittent fasting is, how it works, and the research behind it. You'll learn why this strategy is especially pertinent to and advantageous for women over 50.
- **Tailoring to Your Life:** We recognize that no two lives are the same. We'll walk you through the process of customizing intermittent fasting to fit your particular lifestyle and tastes because of this. We can accommodate your needs regardless of whether you have a demanding schedule, certain dietary restrictions, or other factors.
- **Practical Guidance:** You'll receive information on how to start intermittent fasting, including how to prepare mentally and physically, how to schedule meals, and how to establish goals. We want your trip to go as smoothly as possible.
- **Nutrition Insights:** Learn which foods to eat and which to stay away from while you're fasting, as well as a range of mouthwatering menu options that fit your intermittent fasting objectives.

- Maximising Health Benefits: We'll discuss how intermittent fasting may help you lose weight, have more energy, and have better cognitive function. You'll discover how using intermittent fasting may be a powerful tool for reaching your wellness and health goals.
- Hormonal Balance and Ageing: A woman's life is constantly changing due to hormones, particularly during and after menopause. We'll talk about how achieving hormonal balance with intermittent fasting might help you age gracefully.
- Overcoming Difficulties: Intermittent fasting may be difficult, especially when it comes to coping with hunger and cravings and navigating social settings. We'll provide solutions for overcoming them and staying on course.
- Exercise Integration: Discover effective ways to include exercise into your intermittent fasting plan, as well as advice on how to design a fitness regimen that supports your fasting schedule and enhances general health.
- Long-Term Success: A major goal of intermittent fasting is to maintain its

advantages over time. We'll provide pointers on maintaining consistency, keeping tabs on your development, and acknowledging your successes.

- Real-Life Success Stories: Throughout the manual, you'll read motivational testimonies from actual women over 50 who have adopted intermittent fasting and seen significant changes. These tales provide inspiration and support materials.
- Expert Insights: You'll learn from specialists in the fields of nutrition and health in addition to real-life anecdotes. They'll answer frequently asked questions and provide professional advice to make your intermittent fasting experience better.
- Additional Resources: To broaden your understanding, consult the appendix's list of helpful websites, example menus, and a dictionary.

Chapter 1

The Basics of Intermittent Fasting

The practice of limiting your eating window on a daily, weekly, or monthly basis is known as intermittent fasting. This method's basic tenet is that by cutting down on the amount of time you spend eating, you're giving your body more time to thoroughly digest food, store nutrients, and repair itself before the next mealtime. This not only motivates individuals to make better dietary choices but also offers other health advantages.

Understanding Intermittent Fasting

An eating pattern called intermittent fasting involves alternating between eating and fasting times.

The timing of your meal is more important than the specific things you should consume, according to this advice.

There are several strategies for implementing intermittent fasting, all of which divide the day or week into eating and fasting windows.

Most individuals already "fast" when they sleep each day. Simply making that fast a bit longer might result in intermittent fasting.

The theory behind intermittent fasting is that by limiting our intake, our bodies will more rapidly and effectively use their fat reserves as an energy source. Although glucose from carbs is our most direct fuel source, when glucose isn't available, we turn to fat for energy. When people are food-deprived, this occurs much more often. We can store fat indefinitely.

There are many different methods for intermittent fasting. There isn't a "perfect" fasting schedule, so yours should be based on what works best for you.

One strategy is to fast every day for a certain period, often 12 hours or more. Each night, the typical individual sleeps for roughly 7 hours, which counts toward the required fasting period. You might easily establish a daily fast to boost your body's ability to burn fat if you don't eat after supper. If you often eat at night, this sort of fasting can be beneficial for you.

Alternate-day fasting is another kind of intermittent fasting. Here, you may eat anything you want five to six days a week and choose one or two days to fast. It is advised to drink water and broth during such fasting days to prevent dehydration. For someone whose work schedule may be very hectic sometimes and prevents them from regularly eating, this form of fasting may be useful.

The Science of Fasting

The planet is expanding in size. Although it's a global tendency, the United States does a particularly good job of illustrating it. According to official figures, over three times as many US people than in 1980 and earlier decades were obese as of 2018 (42%) – a figure. Rising incidence of significant health issues including diabetes, atherosclerosis, heart attacks, and strokes are a result of this.

American adults' increased calorie consumption is one factor contributing to all this weight gain. According to national data, between the early 1970s and 2010, daily calorie consumption increased by around 200 calories. Another is that more people are snacking than before. In 2010, US individuals consumed roughly 20% more calories per day as snacks than they had in the early 1970s, and many no longer eat the recommended three meals a day. In a 2015 survey of 156 US people, it was shown that the majority ate more than four times each day on average, and some even up to fifteen times.

However, more scientists are beginning to believe that more than mindless grazing is to blame for the rise in obesity rates. Timing is important as well since we often eat when we shouldn't and don't allow our bodies enough time to recover.

Dominic D'Agostino, a neuroscientist at the University of South Florida who focuses on how diet affects the brain, claims that eating small, frequent meals throughout the day and night was not how we evolved. People instead developed to cope with frequent fasts: We relied on hunting and gathering until the advent of agriculture, which occurred approximately 12,000 years ago, and often had to be done on an empty stomach. According to D'Agostino, "periodic intermittent fasting is hard-wired" in humans.

Studies are beginning to show that eating habits have an impact on body weight and health. The literature reveals important potential benefits from fasting every other day or so, or from eating only when we would normally be awake, within a window of 12 hours or less, a practice known as time-restricted eating, although the research is still inconsistent, heavily animal-dependent, and frequently difficult to parse.

Such behaviors, which have gained thousands of adherents and are sometimes referred to as "intermittent fasting," are said to help prevent obesity and may change the body's metabolism in beneficial ways.

Benefits and Risk for Women Over 50

Numerous symptoms and disorders that might make you seem older than 50 have been demonstrated to have lower risks when intermittent fasting is practiced.

What, I hear you ask? Let's see, then.

The synthesis of sex hormones decreases as women age. Our total metabolism, including insulin resistance, fat storage, cholesterol metabolism, inflammatory regulation, hunger and satiety signals, and skin and sexual health, are significantly influenced by these hormones. As they decline, it may cause:

- changes in skin and hair
- sore joints
- loss of muscle mass and bone density (which increases the risk of falls and broken bones)
- more difficulty keeping a steady weight (ever wonder why losing weight at 50 is more difficult than 25? You have, of course; who hasn't? Less effective at equally spreading fat (it tends to gather mostly around your belly, which is one reason for this)
- heightened risk of diabetes, high blood pressure, and heart disease

To counteract such effects, intermittent fasting may be beneficial:

You have a lower chance of heart disease, high blood pressure, and diabetes if you lose weight or decrease your body fat, improve your blood sugar management, lower your blood pressure, and reduce inflammation.

These advantages are most readily attained when you combine intermittent fasting with healthier eating and exercise routines, which in turn result in extra health advantages including bolstering your bones and joints, enhancing your balance, and restoring the radiance to your skin and hair.

Risks associated with intermittent fasting for older women

We've discussed all the potential advantages of intermittent fasting for women over 50, but there are also concerns.

These are some of the dangers:

- Low blood sugar, lightheadedness, and weakness
- Nutrient shortages
- Muscle mass loss
- Enhanced risk of osteoporosis

With a healthy diet full of whole foods and frequent exercise, many of these risks may be decreased. If you begin fasting and have any adverse effects or health changes that alarm you, see your doctor right away to be safe.

Chapter 2

Adapting Intermittent Fasting to Your Lifestyle

Fasting is a traditional food restriction practice that has gained popularity due to its many advantages for longevity, health, and weight loss.

Although it may seem inconceivable, we are returning to the hunter-gatherer lifestyle that required ancient humans to endure days of continuous fasting.

However, fasting continues to be a tough dietary adjustment that is hard to fit into the hectic contemporary lifestyle. You may adjust and keep fasting as a part of your lifestyle with the aid of this advice.

Selecting the Appropriate Fasting Window

When you first start, choosing when and how to fast is not an easy decision. Here are some pointers for picking the ideal fasting window.

You need to consider your day as a whole first. When do you believe the best times are to eat and when do you believe the best times are to fast?

Given that the majority of us have 9 to 5 jobs and sleep at night, this question could sound absurd. Your fasting and eating windows will be quite different if you work in various time zones or on different shifts, however.

There are several approaches to IF. You are far more likely to be able to put the important techniques you need to succeed with IF into practice and sustain them if you are aware of what to anticipate beforehand and have developed a plan to accommodate the eating and fasting times into your calendar.

The most typical IF kinds are listed below:

- **16:8**

The 16:8 window is the most often used IF strategy because many who use it think it is sustainable, manageable, and maybe a practical approach to reducing weight and improving general health*. The idea is that as long as you fast for 16 hours each day, you are free to eat anything you want for the other 8 hours.

The recommendation is typically to eat between 10:00 a.m. and 6:00 p.m. and then refrain from eating for the rest of the day, including the night and the next morning. Of course, you are 'allowed' to change these times to fit your schedule as long as you adhere to the 16 hours of uninterrupted fasting.

- **14.10 hours of fasting**

This alternative is similar to the previous one in that it just calls for a 14-hour fast each day. Some advantages of fasting, such as increased autophagy, may be lost, but we'll cover this in more detail in a later post.

- **12:12 Fasting, sometimes referred to as an overnight fast.**

An overnight fast is another alternative if a 14-hour fast feels too lengthy for you or if you sometimes enjoy a late meal or an early morning.

This fast lasts just 12 hours, not the usual 14 hours. One of the goals of fasting, regulating insulin levels, is achieved by the body using all of its glucose stores in under 12 hours, according to research. Even though the outcomes will be milder than those of a lengthier fast, the overnight fast is often simple to complete.

- **5:2**

Another well-liked strategy is to eat as much as you like five days a week while restricting yourself to 500 calories on the other two. Most individuals find this method effective because it gives them the choice to pick their two weekly fasting days and allows them to fit them around activities.

- **One Meal a Day (OMAD)**

When you observe a full-day fast, you will only have one meal every day. Again, this is an extremely difficult tactic that can cause women's hormones to shift. Many individuals attempt to just eat once a day, but they consume a lot of coffee or diet drinks to stave off hunger, which may also be harmful.

- **Alternate Day Fasting**

Eating every other day while on an alternate-day fast is quite effective for shedding pounds. The drawback of alternate-day fasting is that it doesn't seem to significantly reduce hunger over time, which makes it unlikely to be a long-term strategy*.

- **Prolonged Fasting**

Longer than 24-hour fasts are considered to be prolonged. Some individuals even observe 21-day fasts! Long-term fasts offer several advantages, including bettering blood sugar regulation11, which helps the body enter a deeper stage of healing. It's important to note that before starting any protracted fasts, a doctor should be contacted to make sure it's appropriate for each individual.

You have it now! Choose the times when you can fast and eat, and then try it. As you go on your IF journey, you may, of course, also change your windows.

How to Make Intermittent Fasting Work for Your Schedule

Any weight reduction program that is both successful AND long-lasting has to be flexible.

Any diet must include some degree of flexibility to be sustained over the long run. You've undoubtedly heard about intermittent fasting by this point. Fasting sometimes may considerably enhance discipline. You'll be able to live a healthier lifestyle overall if you learn how to practice mindful eating and teach your body to grow accustomed to postponing pleasure. Although this diet works well for weight loss, some individuals have trouble sticking to the plan. A more adaptable kind of intermittent fasting has been created as a result. Read on to find out how to make flexible intermittent fasting work for you and start losing weight right now if you need a more flexible weight loss strategy.

A fasting diet not only limits the overall amount of calories you will take each day but also mandates that you consume all of them within a certain window of time each day. You are required under traditional intermittent fasting to consume those calories throughout the same period each day. This is often an 8-hour timeframe, such as 11 a.m. to 7 p.m.

For two key reasons, flexible intermittent fasting is fantastic. First of all, you do not need to follow the same eating window each day. People whose jobs or school schedules change often would appreciate this. Second, the flexible method enables you to ingest some calories, such as those from a drink or a small snack, even when you are fasting. By doing so, you can keep your blood sugar levels stable and prevent weakness and dizziness.

Remember that even if you decide to eat while you're fasting, those calories must still count towards your daily caloric requirement to lose weight.

Making flexible intermittent fasting effective for you is not all that different from making classic intermittent fasting effective. Both, as previously mentioned, need a daily calorie deficit, which will be achieved via a set eating window. Flexible intermittent fasting is much simpler to implement since you may modify it to meet your hectic schedule!

It may be challenging to wait until 11 or 12 to have your first meal, for example, if you work early in the morning. A little snack may keep you satisfied until the start of your actual eating window. Additionally, being able to adjust your feeding window would be quite beneficial if your schedule varies from day to day. Additionally, if you prefer your "coffee with cream" as I do, you may still have a cup in the morning without violating the law!

It will be simpler than ever to follow the plan since you may modify your window to meet your schedule for each day. You will lose weight as long as you consume fewer calories than you burn off via exercise. Because calories in vs. calories out always prevails, there is no magic window. It is not better to consume all of your meals in the morning than at night.

There are a few steps you can take to make flexible intermittent fasting effective for you, regardless of when you've planned your window for the day.

- **Create a Weekly Schedule**

Making a plan might help to keep you on track if you make the effort to do so. Invest some effort in scheduling your eating windows if you know that your job or school schedule will be unpredictable for the forthcoming week. You can follow the plan if you are prepared for the week.

- **Prepare Your Meals in Advance**

It is impossible to emphasize the advantages and significance of having ready-made meals available. You want to be prepared with a nutritious meal when it's time to break your fast so you can start eating right away! Lack of preparation increases your likelihood of stumbling and making poor decisions. Make sure to prepare meals for at least three days in advance.

- **Consume A Lot of Water**

You will experience hunger when fasting, particularly in the beginning. If you're used to having breakfast every morning at 7 a.m. and suddenly have to wait until 11 a.m., you'll be tempted to eat.

While flexible fasting permits the occasional nibble, it is not a good habit to develop. You shouldn't break your fast at an early hour every day. If not, you aren't fasting. Having said that, drinking water will generally suffice you for as long as it takes you to have your first meal.

In addition to accelerating your metabolism, drinking plenty of water will fill you up so that you won't feel hungry. Set a goal to consume at least 64 ounces of liquid every day, but feel free to consume even more!

- **Stick to It**

Time is the most important thing to remember. Although you won't lose weight right away, after a few weeks of being in a calorie deficit, the pounds will start to melt away! Your body may need some time to get used to the new routine, but once it does, you'll start burning fat like crazy!

Flexible intermittent fasting is an option for beginners since it is less limiting than the other methods. But keep in mind that not every diet is suitable for everyone. The success of a weight reduction program is significantly influenced by your schedule and personal preferences. If used correctly, this method of weight reduction may be a very powerful tool. It may help you save money, time, and even energy.

Intermittent fasting may not be appropriate for you if you have diabetes or have trouble controlling your blood sugar. It is strongly advised that you consult your doctor before making any dietary changes.

Common Errors to Avoid

- **Not Choosing the Right Intermittent Fasting Plan**

Since everyone has a distinct body type, not every intermittent fasting regimen will be effective for them. What works for some people may not be as effective for you.

Therefore, the most crucial component focuses on choosing an IF plan that suits your lifestyle, schedule, and objectives. If you can't discover a schedule that works for you and complements your way of life, you'll probably give up on it too soon.

- **Not Consuming Enough When Breaking a Fast**

Many individuals do not understand the distinction between intermittent fasting and dieting, which often results in futile efforts to lose weight. People believe that to get benefits from their diets, they must go on strict fasts throughout their eating window. However, this approach is not only harmful but also unsuccessful.

Contrarily, intermittent fasting enables you to eat as you like within a predetermined window of time. Your body may take a vacation from continually processing food if you eat in this manner.

Lean muscle is necessary for your body to operate efficiently and to continue burning calories even when at rest. Lean muscle is broken down for energy when you don't eat enough during a fast and for a long time. This may be harmful over the long term. Your metabolism may be slowed by the breakdown of muscles, which may lead to tiredness and muscular loss.

These are undesirable results, which is one excellent reason to quit calorie restriction when conducting intermittent fasting. Additionally, after a protracted period of diet restriction, you can start binge eating, which would erase all the benefits of dieting.

Consume enough food to maintain a healthy level of energy, and don't forget to raise your protein intake. Consume protein following your body's requirements to prevent muscle waste and weariness.

- **Overeating After Breaking a Fast**

Hunger is difficult to tolerate, as anybody who has ever been on a diet will attest. This is particularly true if you're attempting to follow a diet that calls for you to fast for extended periods, like intermittent fasting.

However, it's crucial to avoid the desire to overeat when you eventually have a meal. Overeating may rapidly reverse whatever weight reduction you've made and cause unpleasant side effects like bloating and indigestion.

If you want to reduce weight, you need to understand the hormone ghrelin. After a fast, ghrelin makes you feel hungry and makes you more hungry. Ghrelin surges and makes you feel hungrier than before when you overeat, which may swiftly result in weight gain and halt progress.

Eat a light, healthful meal after breaking your fast to stave off hunger and avoid overindulging.

- **Choosing the Wrong Foods During Your Eating Window**

You don't get the right to eat whatever comes your way within your eating window when intermittent fasting. It's important to pay attention to the meals you consume throughout your eating window. Sugary beverages and processed carbohydrates might raise your insulin levels, which can counteract the advantages of fasting.

You won't lose weight if you consume processed meals during intermittent fasting; in fact, you could gain weight. Other health issues including diabetes, heart disease, and high blood pressure may also be brought on by eating junk food.

Instead, concentrate on eating wholesome, healthful meals that will make you feel energized and fulfilled. Fruits, veggies, and lean protein are all excellent alternatives. A low-calorie whey protein supplement might help you meet your protein requirements if you're a busy bee.

Additionally, if you're craving something sweet, try some nuts or some fruit. You can only fully profit from intermittent fasting by making wise decisions when you are eating.

- **Not Consuming Enough Water**

Whether or whether you are fasting, water is an essential component of any weight reduction diet. While fasting, drinking enough water will help you feel satiated for longer and less inclined to eat. Additionally, when your body is properly hydrated, it will perform better all around.

According to medical experts, you should consume at least eight glasses of water each day. When you are fasting, you must do this. You may always try other unsweetened drinks like green tea or herbal teas if water isn't your cup of tea (no pun intended).

Black coffee has been known to cause dehydration in certain individuals, although moderate doses are OK sometimes. Take an additional glass of water with each cup of coffee.

- **Taking Your Fast Break Unknowingly**

The phrase "clean fast" confounds a lot of people. Water, black coffee, and unsweetened tea are the only things that may be consumed during a clean fast. When fasting, it's important to be mindful of what you're drinking since many popular drinks hide calories and carbohydrates.

The majority of "diet" or "zero-calorie" foods often include a lot of artificial sweeteners, some of which may break your fast, even if they claim to have almost no calories.

During your fasting window, drinking anything other than water, black coffee, or unsweetened tea will break your fast and prevent you from reaping the advantages of intermittent fasting. This may be annoying, particularly if you're attempting too fast to experience advantages like ketosis and autophagy.

Check the labels before drinking a beverage during a fast to determine whether the contents include any unstated calories or nutrients that might end your fast.

- **Not Exercising While Fasting**

Physical exercise is essential whether you want to enhance your health or reduce weight. Exercise increases insulin sensitivity and speeds up metabolism in addition to burning calories. These are all essential components of a healthy lifestyle and effective weight reduction.

If you don't exercise during intermittent fasting, you lose out on additional benefits including calorie-burning and a boosted metabolism, all of which are necessary for losing weight.

Since your body requires muscle tissue for energy, fasting may also cause muscle loss. A decline in metabolism follows this loss of bulk. Strengthen your muscles often to prevent this; over time, you could also experience healthy weight gain as a result.

Maintain or begin an exercise regimen during intermittent fasting to help burn fat and enhance health. Exercise for at least 30 minutes every day of the week; even moderately intense activities, including brisk walking, cycling, swimming, or light training, are sufficient.

- **Having Dinner too Late**

Many individuals feel that later in the day, they have more energy and concentration, thus they often eat supper later than normal. Even though it may not seem like a major matter, it can interfere with the body's circadian rhythms, which can cause several health issues.

For instance, eating late at night might disrupt your ability to fall asleep and remain asleep by interfering with your body's normal sleep cycle. It may also impede digestion, resulting in indigestion and other gastrointestinal problems.

So eat supper early to promote digestion and sleep, all of which are crucial for losing weight.

Chapter 3

Getting Started with Intermittent Fasting

Are you interested in learning more about the benefits of intermittent fasting for your health and well-being? Look nowhere else! This thorough book will go deeply into the realm of intermittent fasting and provide you with all the details you need to begin making this effective lifestyle adjustment.

Mental Preparation

If your mind is ready, fasting will be a lot simpler.

Being gentle to yourself and not comparing your experience to others are the two most crucial pieces of fasting bits of advice to keep in mind. Several intricate, ever-changing elements determine how easy or difficult you find fasting. A friend's fasting experience is something you may listen to and learn from, but you shouldn't compare it to your own. Nobody in the world is exactly like you, therefore any objectives, challenges, or triumphs you experience cannot be compared to those of others.

- Setting an intention . Are you aiming to relieve your gastrointestinal system, control your blood sugar, encourage autophagy (cell recycling), shed some pounds, show yourself you can do it, or anything else? Your fast will go a lot more smoothly if you know why you're doing it and keep yourself reminded of it sometimes, whether it's by posting notes on your mirror, setting up reminders, or getting unexpected messages.
- Set a time limit for how long you want to fast and mentally be ready for it with your objective clearly in mind. Will you observe a 14-hour fast? 36? Longer? If you have never fasted before, you may want to begin by skipping one or two meals to prove to your body and yourself that you are capable of doing so. Set a longer target once you've done one or a few short fasts. If you're planning a lengthy fast, have diabetes, an eating issue, are on medication, or have any health condition, you should speak with a doctor before choosing a target.

- Keep in mind that your path and your objectives are unique to you and should allow for some flexibility. Consider extending if you feel excellent after exceeding your 24-hour objective. Similarly to this, you may need to change your objective to something less challenging if you start to feel nauseous or dizzy just halfway through it. Pay attention to your body and take your special trip.
- Inform your friends, fast with others, or join a group (Redmond Fasting is our favorite). When you fast, you could feel wonderful after 18 hours, hungry after 26, and re energized after 31. Fasting with friends or having them support you will help you get through the challenging times. If you have concerns or unanticipated symptoms, a community may also be a useful resource. However, a fan club is optional, and some individuals would rather keep their objectives a secret. There is no right or incorrect strategy.

Meal Planning and Grocery Shopping

The lack of dietary limits and merely time constraints for eating are two of the most alluring aspects of intermittent fasting.

Even said, a lot of individuals who fast intermittently also follow a diet or just wish to know how to lead a healthy lifestyle.

Probably the reason you're on this page is to find a precise intermittent fasting food list from which to organize your meals. Before making any major dietary changes, you must first speak with a qualified medical professional.IF isn't appropriate for everyone, so talk to a qualified specialist about it.

This post's objective is to present you with examples of items you may eat as part of a diverse diet while you engage in intermittent fasting; it is not meant to provide any professional or medical advice.

When engaging in intermittent fasting, it is a good idea to follow the following recommendations for healthy eating in general:

- Eat foods that have undergone the least amount of processing when you are eating most of the time.
- Consume a diet that is balanced and includes lean proteins, fruits, vegetables, whole grains, and healthy fats.
- Prepare delectable dishes that you will like eating.
- Eat gently and thoroughly until you are full.

Realistic Goal-Setting

To make sure that intermittent fasting (IF) for women over 50 is in line with their health, way of life, and particular requirements, it is crucial to set realistic objectives. Although intermittent fasting may enhance metabolic health and help you control your weight, it's important to proceed with care, particularly as you become older. Here are some recommendations for creating practical IF goals:

- Speak with a Healthcare Professional: It's critical to speak with your doctor or a certified dietitian before beginning any fasting program. They may assess your present state of health, existing illnesses, and prescription drugs to establish if intermittent fasting is risk-free and appropriate for you.

- Recognise the Various IF Techniques: Several methods, including the 16/8 technique, the 5:2 diet, and alternate-day fasting, fall under the umbrella of intermittent fasting. Every technique has a unique set of guidelines and fasting times. Pick the one that best suits your interests and lifestyle.

- Begin Gradually: It's a good idea to ease into intermittent fasting if you're new to it. Start with a less severe fasting regimen and progressively widen it as your body gets used to it. For instance, start with a 12-hour overnight fast and then increase it by an hour every few days until you reach the fasting window of your choice.

- Watch your Calorie Intake: Intermittent fasting should not be used as an excuse to overeat while you are eating. Keep an eye on your food intake's nutritional value and portion proportions. Emphasize nutrient-dense foods like whole grains, lean meats, fruits, and vegetables.

- Remain Hydrated: During your fasting times, be sure to remain hydrated by consuming water, herbal teas, or other non-caloric liquids. Exhaustion and pain are consequences of dehydration.

- Pay Attention to your Body's Signals; if necessary, modify your fasting plan. If you feel excessively hungry, lightheaded, or in any other pain, think about changing your fasting window or technique.
- Establish Reasonable Weight Reduction Targets: If managing your weight is one of your objectives, strive for a steady decrease of between 0.5 and 1 pound each week. This normally calls for a calorie deficit during your eating windows, but rather than a diet of severe restriction, it should be accomplished with a balanced diet.
- Place a Priority on Overall Health: While losing weight may be a goal, don't ignore other facets of health. By combining stress management, regular physical exercise, and a good night's sleep into your routine, you may improve your entire well-being, including your mental health.
- Track Progress and Make Adjustments: Keep a notebook or use a tracking tool to keep track of your fasting pattern, meals, and overall feelings. Review your

objectives often and make any necessary changes in light of your experiences and health results.

- Have Patience and Flexibility: Achieving health and fitness objectives might take some time, particularly as we become older. Be kind to yourself and flexible in your approach so that it may be adjusted to your body's shifting requirements.

Chapter 4

Selecting the Best Foods

There are several popular weight-loss diets, but is intermittent fasting one of them? With celebrities like Jennifer Aniston, Molly Sims, and Kate Walsh advocating the diet, intermittent fasting has gained attention recently. But here's the thing ask any of them and they'll tell you that intermittent fasting isn't a diet but rather a way of life that involves time-restricted eating patterns and that promotes wellbeing and results in weight loss as well as improved health.

But is intermittent fasting beneficial for women over 50, or is it simply another diet or "detox" fad? Find out by reading on! Stick to wholesome whole meals and drinks throughout mealtimes to maximize the possible health advantages of your diet.

Including enough nutrient-dense foods in your diet can help you maintain a healthy weight. Attempt to include a variety of whole foods at each meal, such as:

- Fruits: Apples, Bananas, Berries, Oranges, Peaches, Pears, Tomatoes, etc.

- Vegetables: Broccoli, Brussels sprouts, Cauliflower, Cucumbers, Leafy Greens, etc.
- Whole grains include barley, buckwheat, quinoa, rice, oats, and others.
- Healthy fats include avocados and olive oil.
- Foods high in protein include eggs, fish, beans, meat, poultry, nuts, and seeds.
- Even when fasting, staying hydrated and controlling your hunger may be accomplished by consuming calorie-free drinks like water, unsweetened tea, and coffee.

Nutrient-Rich Foods for Women Over 50

For women over 50 to sustain general health, particularly during intermittent fasting, nutrient-rich diets are crucial. Some people may benefit from intermittent fasting, but it's important to make sure you're receiving all the nutrients you need, particularly as you become older. Here is a list of meals high in nutrients and things to keep in mind for women over 50 who fast intermittently:

- Leafy Greens: Kale, Swiss chard, collard greens and spinach are all great sources of antioxidants, vitamins, and minerals.
- Lean Proteins: Include lean protein sources including fowl, fish, tofu, tempeh, and lentils in your diet. Protein improves general health and helps keep muscles strong.
- Fruits: Apples, pears, citrus fruits, berries, and citrus fruits all include vitamins, fiber, and antioxidants. Additionally, they have fewer calories than several other fruits.
- Whole Grains: To give necessary carbs and fiber for long-lasting energy, choose whole grains like quinoa, brown rice, oats, and whole wheat pasta.
- Nuts and Seeds: Almonds, walnuts, chia seeds, and flaxseeds are abundant in omega-3 fatty acids as well as fiber and good fats.
- Dairy or Dairy Alternatives: For calcium and vitamin D, choose low-fat or plant-

based alternatives such as almond or soy milk.

- Probiotic Foods: Fermented foods like kimchi and sauerkraut, as well as yogurt, promote gut health and may improve general well-being.
- Fatty Fish: Sardines, salmon, and mackerel are full of omega-3 fatty acids, which may help fight inflammation and promote heart health.
- Foods High in Calcium: Leafy greens, dairy products, and plant-based milk with added calcium may all support bone health.
- Iron-Rich Foods: To maintain appropriate iron consumption, which is essential for energy and oxygen transport in the body, include lean red meat, poultry, beans, and fortified cereals.
- Vitamin D: Sunlight exposure and fortified foods like orange juice and cereals may help keep vitamin D levels in check, which is crucial for bone health.
- Hydration: Drink plenty of water, herbal teas, and low-sugar drinks to improve digestion and general health.

It's critical to have a variety of these nutrient-dense meals in your eating window while doing intermittent fasting to satisfy your nutritional demands. Here are some other things to think about:

- Consult a Healthcare Professional: To make sure a fasting regimen is safe for you before beginning, particularly if you have underlying medical concerns, speak with a healthcare professional or registered dietitian.
- Hydration: To keep hydrated when fasting, consume adequate water.
- Multivitamin Supplements: In certain circumstances, a multivitamin supplement may be required to fill any potential nutritional shortages, although it's always preferable to get nutrients through whole meals.
- Monitor How You Feel: Be aware of how you feel physically. If you encounter negative side effects or pain when fasting intermittently, think about changing your fasting schedule or seeking advice from a specialist.

Foods to Stay Away From During Fasting Periods

Several items should not be consumed when following an intermittent fasting plan. Avoid foods that are rich in calories and have high levels of salt, sugar, and fat. They won't satisfy you after a fast and can make you feel more ravenous, according to Maciel. Additionally, they provide very little to no nutrition.

Avoid these foods if you want to follow a healthy intermittent eating plan:

- Snack chips
- Microwave popcorn.

You should also stay away from meals that include a lot of added sugar. According to Maciel, processed sugar is nutritionally worthless and just provides sweet, empty calories, which is not what you want if you're occasionally fasting. Due to how quickly the sugar metabolizes, he claims that eating them will make you hungry.

You should stay away from the following sugary foods if you're intermittent fasting:

Cookies.

- Candy.
- Cakes.
- Ketchup and BBQ sauce.
- Fruit Juice.
- Sugary granola and cereal.

Recipes and Meal Suggestions

The kinds of recipes and meal options you choose will depend on your particular fasting window and nutritional preferences. Intermittent fasting may be a flexible way to eat. Here are some menu suggestions for those who fast intermittently:

16/8 Fasting (16 hours of fasting, followed by 8 hours of eating):

- **Breakfast**: Greek yogurt topped with fruit and honey.
- Eggs scrambled with tomatoes and spinach.
- Banana slices and almonds on top of oatmeal.
- **Lunch**: Grilled chicken salad with mixed greens and vinaigrette dressing .
- Bowl of quinoa, black beans, avocado, and salsa.
- A stir-fry of vegetables and tofu.
- **Dinner**: Baked salmon with quinoa and steamed broccoli.
- Spaghetti squash topped with marinara and served with roasted asparagus on the side.
- Lean beef or turkey chili served with mixed greens on the side.
- **Snacks** (during the eating window): Almonds or a combination of nuts.
- Cucumber slices with hummus.
- Cottage cheese with pieces of pineapple.

5:2 Fasting (2 days apart with extremely low-calorie intake):

- On days when you're fasting, try to eat meals that have between 500 and 600 calories, such as:
- Vegetable soup with a modest serving of lean protein.
- Baked sweet potato with steaming veggies on the side.
- A small salad including grilled chicken or tofu as a protein source.
- Consume balanced, nutrient-rich meals as suggested in the preceding response on days when you typically eat.

Alternate -Day Fasting:

- Consider low-calorie dishes on days when you're fasting, such as a substantial salad with greens, vegetables, and lean protein.
- A protein-packed smoothie prepared with berries, spinach, and unsweetened almond milk.
- A soup made with a lot of veggies and broth.
- On days when you aren't fasting, eat a variety of healthy, whole foods.

The Warrior Diet (20 hours of fasting, followed by 4 hours of eating):

- When planning your 4-hour eating window, focus on filling, nutrient-dense meals like
- A large salad with grilled chicken or salmon.
- A serving of tofu, mixed veggies, and brown rice or quinoa.
- Stir-fried vegetables or lean meat with brown rice.

"OMAD" or "One Meal a Day"

- Consume your complete day's worth of calories in a single, nutritious meal that is well-balanced and has all the necessary elements.
- For instance, a dish with lean protein (chicken, fish, or tofu), plenty of veggies, a portion of nutritious grains (brown rice or quinoa), and healthy fats (avocado or olive oil).

Chapter 5

Maximising Health Benefits

You should adhere to several important rules and take particular aspects into account to maximize the health advantages of intermittent fasting:

- Consult a Healthcare Professional: Before beginning any fasting program, particularly if you have underlying medical concerns or are taking medication, speak with a healthcare professional or qualified dietitian. They may provide you with tailored advice depending on your particular situation.
- Select the Appropriate Fasting Method: There are a variety of intermittent fasting strategies available. Choose the one that best suits your tastes and way of life. The 16/8 technique, 5:2 fasting, alternate-day fasting, the Warrior Diet, and OMAD (One Meal a Day) are examples of popular approaches.
- Pay Attention to Nutrient Quality: Prioritising nutrient-dense meals within your eating window is crucial when

fasting. Include a mix of whole grains, lean meats, fruits, vegetables, healthy fats, dairy products, or dairy substitutes in your diet to make sure you're receiving all the vitamins and minerals you need.

- Maintain Hydration: To maintain hydration when fasting, consume lots of water, herbal teas, and other non-caloric liquids. Water intake has to be right for general health and well-being.
- Regulate Portion Sizes: Watch your portion sizes, particularly after a fast. The advantages of fasting may be lost if you consume too much within your eating window. Control your portion sizes and pay attention to your body's hunger signals.
- Stay Away from Highly Processed Foods: Limit the amount of processed and sugary meals you eat. These may cause unhealthy blood sugar spikes and crashes, which can be particularly troublesome during fasting.
- Include Fibre: Foods high in fiber, such as fruits, vegetables, whole grains, and legumes, may make you feel satisfied for longer periods and promote digestive health.

- Incorporate Protein: Adding enough protein to your meals will help you maintain lean muscle mass and increase satiety.
- Monitor Your Health: Keep tabs on your vital signs, including weight, blood pressure, and blood sugar levels. This may assist you in determining how intermittent fasting will affect your health and help you make the required corrections.
- Exercise Regularly: Combine regular exercise with intermittent fasting for better overall health and weight control. Create a proper workout regimen by speaking with a fitness expert.
- Sleep and Stress Management: Give excellent sleep and stress-reduction strategies a high priority since they have a substantial impact on general health and may enhance the advantages of intermittent fasting.
- Be Patient and Flexible: Keep in mind that it could take some time for your body to adjust to intermittent fasting. Be patient with the procedure and adapt your strategy as necessary.
- Consider Supplements: You may need to take supplements, such as vitamin D,

vitamin B12, or omega-3 fatty acids, to make sure you're fulfilling all of your nutritional needs, depending on your dietary preferences and particular needs.

- Regular Check-ups: Arrange frequent visits with your doctor to monitor your health and go through any issues or modifications to your fasting schedule.

Numerous health advantages, including better metabolic function, improved weight control, and possible advantages for longer life, may be obtained by intermittent fasting. However, it's crucial to approach it attentively and make sure it satisfies your unique requirements and objectives in terms of health. Before making any substantial dietary or fasting-related changes, always get medical advice.

Increasing Your Energy

The lesser-known advantage of intermittent fasting is supposed to be an increase in energy, in addition to weight reduction. Our metabolism cycles through the process of converting carbs into blood sugar when we eat multiple times

throughout the day. It eventually becomes energy or is stored in cells for later use. Your energy and mental performance decline as a result of the body's consumption or storage of sugar, which causes blood sugar to fall. This sends out a "hunger signal," presumably causing us to eat, and the cycle repeats. Our metabolism is stressed by the daylong ups and downs in blood sugar, which lowers our general energy and mental performance.

What makes intermittent fasting different? When fat is used as fuel, it must first be processed into ketones in the liver due to its sluggish rate of digestion. We have more energy and feel better, and our levels of focus and cognitive function are also greater since this process occurs slowly and regularly without any ups and downs.

Where is the catch if having more energy makes accomplishing exercise objectives easier?

Intermittent fasting isn't for everyone, as wonderful as it sounds. Consider it as a new way of life that your body must first get used to. It's typical to first feel low on energy, very hungry, and even lightheaded. The advantages take a few weeks to manifest. Be patient and avoid basing your judgment on how you first feel. Keep going and allow your body time to adjust to your new way of life. You will eventually feel less hungry and more energized when the hormone ghrelin, which affects how you feel about food and when you're full, is produced.

Improving Cognitive Performance

The most prevalent dementia condition and leading cause of mortality is Alzheimer's disease. The hallmark is neurofibrillary tangles, which are aberrant tau protein aggregates, and beta-amyloid (A) neuritic plaques, which cause cognitive impairment, including memory loss and learning challenges. Even though it is advised to eat frequently for excellent cognition, researchers have shown that intermittent fasting enhances these cognitive capacities. This comprehensive study intends to further explore whether intermittent fasting improves cognitive performance in Alzheimer's disease and if levels of A- and tau-pathology contribute to these improvements. Does intermittent fasting enhance cognitive function in Alzheimer's disease, and if so, does the presence of A and tau pathology explain these improvements in cognition? Three electronic databases—Pubmed, Web of Science, and WorldCat—were searched for publications in the literature, yielding n=744 results. The cognitive tests revealed a tendency towards better learning, memory, and exploratory behavior among people with Alzheimer's disease who intermittently fast. Although contradictory, the impacts on the levels of A and tau pathology raise the potential of a more serious, underlying Alzheimer's disease problem.

Chapter 6

Managing Hormones And Aging Gracefully

Beyond just intermittent fasting, managing hormones and aging gracefully involves a variety of lifestyle choices. The following guidelines and tactics will assist women over 50 in managing their hormones and aging gracefully:

- Prioritize a balanced diet full of entire foods, such as fruits, vegetables, lean meats, whole grains, and healthy fats. These provide vital nutrients for maintaining hormonal balance and good health in general.

- Considerations for Intermittent Fasting: Some people may benefit from intermittent fasting, but it may not be appropriate for everyone. Fasting's effects on hormone levels, energy levels, and general well-being should be particularly watched by women over 50. To be sure it's the best course of action for you, speak with a certified dietitian or healthcare professional.

- Hormone-Healthy Foods: Include cruciferous vegetables (broccoli, cauliflower), flaxseeds, fatty fish (salmon, sardines), and foods high in antioxidants (berries, dark leafy greens) into your diet to promote hormonal balance.
- Protein Intake: Make sure you consume enough protein to assist in the maintenance of muscles and the health of your hormones. Include lean items in your diet, such as tofu, beans, fish, and fowl.
- Omega-3 Fatty Acids: These fats, which may be found in fish, walnuts, and chia seeds, can aid in lowering inflammation and maintaining hormonal balance.
- Fibre: Foods high in fiber, such as whole grains, legumes, and vegetables, may assist with digestion and hormone regulation.
- Hydration: Drink enough water to be well hydrated. To maintain hormonal balance and general health, one must drink enough water.
- Stress Management: Prolonged stress might mess with your hormone levels. Engage in stress-reduction activities or practices like yoga, meditation, or mindful breathing.

- Exercise Regularly: Exercise regularly to maintain muscular mass, boost metabolism, and support hormonal health.
- Adequate Sleep: Give quality sleep a high priority; strive for 7-9 hours per night. Hormone balance and general health depend on sleep.
- Regular Check-ups: Arrange routine check-ups with your doctor to monitor hormone levels and talk about any worries you may have about aging and hormone changes.
- HRT (Hormone Replacement Therapy): When menopause-related hormonal abnormalities are present, a healthcare professional may sometimes advise hormone replacement treatment. With a healthcare expert, go through the pros and cons.
- Skin Care and Sun Protection: To reduce the outward indications of aging, follow a skincare program and protect your skin from sun damage.
- Mental and Emotional Well-being: To promote your general well-being as you age, cultivate a positive outlook, partake in enjoyable activities, and create meaningful social relationships.

- Stay Informed: To make well-informed choices about your well-being, stay current on the most recent studies and advice for women's health and aging.

Balancing Hormones Through Fasting

Your progesterone and estrogen levels fluctuate throughout the menstrual cycle. Gonadotropin-releasing hormone (GnRH) plays a major role in controlling how your hormones rise and decrease.

"GnRH can be very sensitive to environmental factors," says Zumpano. Fasting, for example, prevents the release of the molecules required to boost estrogen and progesterone.

That might have evolutionary roots. Ovulation, the window of your cycle during which you might get pregnant, is brought on by an increase in a few hormones. According to the hypothesis, fasting may cause your body to act as if there is a lack of food and that you may starve to death. These are not the best circumstances for a safe pregnancy. So, to avoid becoming pregnant, your body suppresses ovulation.

It, therefore, reduces your body's levels of estrogen and progesterone, which may lead to a variety of symptoms, such as:

- Modifications in your menstrual cycle, including missed periods.
- Anxiety or melancholy.
- Night sweats and hot flushes.
- Migraines.
- Low libido and sex desire.
- Dry skin.
- Alopecia.
- Acne.
- A sleeping disorder.
- Infertility and palpitations are two symptoms.

How to safely fast for women

Intermittent fasting isn't advised if you're expecting, nursing (chestfeeding), or trying to become pregnant. However, if you're a pre-menopausal woman, you may still be able to benefit from some of the hormone-neutralizing effects of intermittent fasting. However, you need first take a few safety measures.

Not that women should never attempt intermittent fasting. It's that if they step carefully, they'll be better off," Zumpano reiterates.

Don't take things too far.

People approach intermittent fasting in a variety of ways, some more rigorously than others. Some individuals limit their meals to certain times of the day. certain people will eat normally on certain days of the week while drastically cutting down on calories on other days.

According to Zumpano, pre-menopausal females may benefit most from an initial low-intensity intermittent fasting program. I advise beginning with a 12-hour fasting plan. For the majority of individuals, that access point is rather secure.

For instance, you may begin by fasting from 8 p.m. to 8 a.m. every day.

After a week, if everything is going well for you, you may extend it by two hours by adding an hour of fasting on each side, according to Zumpano. You may now fast from 7 p.m. to 9 a.m. if you were previously fasting from 8 p.m. to 8 a.m.

Zumpano advises restricting your food to an eight-hour window and building up to a 16-hour fast overnight. If you're menstruation, be sure to timing it properly to your cycle (keep reading!).

Fast when it matters

Some periods of the month are preferable to others for trying intermittent fasting if you haven't gone through menopause.

If you synchronize your fasting with your cycle, Zumpano says, it will be more successful and produce less hormonal imbalance.

A day or two following the start of your period and a week or so after are better periods to experiment with fasting. You should cut down on your fasting during the two weeks before your menstruation. Two weeks before your period, you're most likely to be ovulating. Your hormones are thus most likely to be impacted by fasting at that period.

The week before your menstruation, avoid fasting. Your body is most susceptible to stress at that time. During that time, estrogen levels fall, which makes the stress hormone cortisol more sensitive. Because of this, the week leading up to your period may include mood changes, poor energy, and an increase in appetite or food cravings.

Slowing Down the Aging Process

Fasting, often known as fad dieting, may assist the body to maintain a healthy balance to some level. However, engaging in prolonged and extreme fasting to lose weight can have negative effects on your general health, with noticeable symptoms showing up on the skin.

New research found that fasting boosts the body's metabolic activity, which further promotes physical wellness and good skin. Additionally, it has anti-aging advantages. In actuality, fad diets like intermittent fasting aid in weight loss and may lengthen life.

In a study by Dr. Takayuki Teruya and a group of researchers from the Okinawa Institute of Science and Technology Graduate University in Japan, the effect of metabolism on skin aging was investigated. According to a study, fasting and calorie restriction improve immunity and metabolism.

Effects on skin health

Our bodies undergo extended starvation when fasting, which causes metabolic alterations. In the absence of food, our body relies on stored fat to produce glucose, which serves as our body's energy source. This process is called gluconeogenesis. The body obtains glucose from substances other than carbohydrates, such as amino acids. Fasting also boosts the levels of purines and pyrimidine in the body, which raises the body's antioxidant capacity and benefits both the general health of the body and the health of the skin.

In layman's terms, good eating and fasting aid in the body's maintenance of a balanced state, which in turn strengthens the metabolism and boosts immunity. The increase in antioxidant levels promotes healthy skin and slows the aging process of the skin. However, eating a good diet following a fasting period slows down skin aging. Therefore, eating regularly and eating well are the keys to having good skin.

Addressing Menopause and Hormonal Changes

You don't want to worry about hormones or managing your weight as you approach your fifties. They continue to be a part of your life, nevertheless. Thankfully, intermittent fasting for women over 50 offers a real chance to support your busy and healthy lifestyle. advantages of intermittent fasting (IF) include advantages for managing and losing weight. Additionally, it helps with hormone balance throughout menopause and perimenopause and promotes healthy aging. Intermittent fasting may help you age gracefully and completely appreciate every minute of your middle years.

Due to its variety of health advantages and the fact that it doesn't limit your dietary options, intermittent fasting has gained popularity in recent years. According to research, fasting may enhance your metabolism and mental health, and perhaps even stave against certain malignancies. Additionally, it may prevent several muscle, nerve, and joint problems that often afflict women over 50.

Menopause and Fasting

When you reach menopause, it has been a year since you last had a period. Your ability to have children is essentially gone. It usually takes place around the age of 50.

In the years after menopause, your estrogen and progesterone levels are quite stable. They remain at a low level and steady.

Because of this, postmenopausal ladies in their 50s, 60s, and beyond may find that intermittent fasting is more beneficial, according to Zumpano. But you should still use caution.

Ovulation and menstruation won't be impacted by intermittent fasting after menopause, according to her. But even after menopause, some women continue to show signs of low hormone levels. Therefore, you should still exercise caution and be vigilant about checking to see whether fasting is resulting in any new symptoms.

Chapter 7

Overcoming Challenges

determining the ideal moment to fast. Think about which one you can miss when deciding which timeframe is the greatest for your fast. Is it breakfast or dinner? It will be more difficult than working from home if you are working in an office or shifts. Be ready to adapt.

Can you achieve success? Yes!

- Adjust your schedule as necessary. Sometimes you can only complete 12:12, but whenever you can, strive to complete 16:8.
- Planning is essential. During your non-fasting hours, prepare your lunch and supper for today and tomorrow.
- Put more emphasis on how you feel and how your clothing fits rather than what the scale says. The inches are what matter.
- Maintain your busyness. You should read, exercise, or plant to divert your attention from eating.
- Be aware of your body. Eat if you're hungry.

- Show patience. It'll take some time.

On this path, never forget to treat yourself with kindness.

Don't give up on yourself or your health even though life occurs, and it's good to change as necessary.

Handling Hunger and Cravings

Intermittent fasting does cause hunger, but probably not in the way you think. If you've ever had a "hanger," or the sensation of being both hungry and furious, you may imagine that this feeling is 10 times worse while fasting. That is not the situation. Most individuals are oblivious to this because they don't let hunger linger for long, if at all; it only lasts for around 20 minutes.

In other circumstances, individuals never experience actual hunger since their appetite keeps them satisfied all the time. The urge to eat, known as an appetite, may be brought on by hormones, senses (such as sights, sounds, and odors), or even emotions like boredom and tension. On the other hand, true hunger is a desire to eat that is accompanied by discomfort and stomach churning. This is a crucial difference to establish since it will enable you to regulate your appetite if you know why you are feeling hungry.

The most crucial concept to grasp is that feeling hungry is normal and that you shouldn't be frightened of it. Although it could feel unpleasant at first, nothing negative will occur. Hunger is a conditioned reaction to a stimulus that may be reconditioned, as Pavlov proved. Have you ever observed, for instance, that hunger pangs occur every day at the same time?

This is because the body has learned to stimulate hunger at regular feeding times since the hormone ghrelin increases in anticipation of a meal. Inventive, huh?

The first few days of fasting are perhaps the most difficult since actual hunger will take some getting used to and your "learned appetite" will tempt you to eat. But there are many methods you may use to calmly ride the hungry wave. To assist you in achieving your fasting objective, I'll go through 7 strategies in this post that may help you control your hunger.

- **Eat a high-fat, low-carb diet.**

Both when you eat and what you consume are crucial. Keep in mind that eating mediocre food is not permitted while you practice intermittent fasting. Use it instead to maximize the benefits of your diet and health.

In between fasts, we advise sticking to high-quality, low-carb, high-fat, and moderate-protein meals. This will help keep blood sugar levels stable, encourage fullness, and make fasting just a little bit easier.

- **Start with a low-carb and high-fat diet.**

Continuing from the previous point, laying the groundwork with a low-carb diet is an excellent method to begin intermittent fasting. Your hunger will have greatly decreased if you become fat acclimated (effectively utilizing fat as fuel instead of glucose), and fasting will come naturally and without effort.

Give yourself at least two weeks to make dietary changes before thinking about incorporating intermittent fasting.

- **Avoid alcohol, lower your stress levels, and obtain a decent night's sleep.**

Alcohol, stress, and lack of sleep all have a significant impact on appetite by interfering with hormone and blood sugar regulation.

By getting more rest, using stress management strategies, and consuming less alcohol, you may avoid these hungry sensations brought on by sugar and hormones.

Make sure your bedroom is cool and well-ventilated, set a regular bedtime that's not too late, block out light and noise, avoid eating three hours before bed, avoid screens and blue light an hour before bed, wind down with a book, and include exercise in your daily routine to improve the quality of your sleep.

Your stress levels will undoubtedly benefit from a restful night's sleep. You may also practice stress-reduction practices like yoga, meditation, exercise, journaling, and therapy for an added boost of serenity and serotonin (the happy hormone).

To avoid irregular hormone and blood sugar levels, try to minimize alcohol intake as much as you can, especially the day before a fast. Naturally, consider low-carb foods in moderation if you do want to consume alcohol.

We'll go into more depth about this in our alcohol guide.

- **Maintain hydration**

Keep yourself hydrated with plenty of water since thirst is sometimes mistaken for hunger. Try to hydrate yourself as soon as you wake up by consuming one to two glasses of water. Aim for around 2-3 liters of water overall each day; exceeding this amount will cause the body to lose vital electrolytes.

Water may aid with actual hunger sensations by providing a bodily feeling of fullness. Water is your tool when fasting, no matter what level of hunger you are feeling.

Try altering the temperature — depending on whether you like warm or chilly water — to make it more tolerable if you have trouble drinking water, particularly in the morning. If it doesn't work, another option is to use sparkling water that has been infused with lemon and mint.

- **Consume salt and replenish electrolytes.**

Electrolyte depletion is a typical and expected reaction to intermittent fasting. As a consequence, despite your efforts to drink plenty of water, you could have a thirst and dry mouth. As previously mentioned, thirst and hunger are often confused, thus these feelings may be painful and make you feel hungry.

Because electrolytes are crucial for health and wellness, we implore you to maintain optimal levels before symptoms appear. You may consume bone broth and salt meals generously during your eating window to replenish electrolytes. A magnesium and potassium supplement, which you may take while fasting, can also be beneficial. Our guide on electrolytes, which will go through everything in greater depth, is available here.

Another excellent approach to clear the palette and quell hunger is with a dash of salt. Use a little amount at a time, dab a few times on your tongue, and wait for it to perform its magic;

soon, the awful coating in your mouth and hunger will be gone.

- **Sip some tea or coffee.**

Freshly prepared black tea or coffee may fill the need left by the absence of nourishment. Like drinking water, a hot beverage will make you feel full but also occupy your "hand to mouth" activity, giving you the impression that you have eaten.

Consider drinking bulletproof coffee, which is coffee with extra fats like butter, coconut oil, MCT oil, and ghee, if you're truly having trouble with hunger and intermittent fasting. As you sustain ketosis and autophagy, two crucial processes that support fasting and its advantages, the fat will keep you satisfied. However, if adding fat to your coffee helps you stay with a fast or makes it simpler for you, I would say it is 100% worth it. For the fasting purist, taking even one calorie will end a fast.

- **Use a distraction**

Plan to work out, participate in extracurricular activities, and visit friends at mealtimes or whenever you feel hungry. Ghrelin levels will spike around mealtimes, as we previously stated, so be ready and make plans to do something enjoyable then. You won't even be aware that ghrelin-induced hunger has arrived and gone since you'll be so busy having fun. By all means, avoid being bored at all costs. As we all know, this is a certain way for hunger to sneak in.

Don't be scared of hunger, but be ready for it. I assure you that hunger won't be as unpleasant as you think. With these methods and suggestions under your belt, you'll be able to put an end to hunger cravings and accomplish your fasting objective in no time. Remember that while fasting alters our conditioned hunger, it becomes easier the more you do it. As you begin to listen to the rhythm of actual hunger rather than appetite, fasting will soon become an instinctual, natural part of your day.

Having said that, you may need to modify your fasting regimen if hunger becomes too intense. Fasting should be manageable, pleasant, and integrated into your daily life. Check out my article from last week where I cover how to fit a fast into your lifestyle for additional information on this.

Social and Emotional Aspects

In particular, as women age, social and emotional factors are essential parts of total wellbeing. Here are some things to think about and approaches for dealing with these aspects:

Social aspects include:

- Keep Social Connections: Keep in touch with friends and family. An important component of mental health is social support, which may also give one a feeling of community.
- Join Social Groups: Look into joining clubs, organizations, or hobby groups that share your interests. You might make new friends and take part in satisfying activities as a result of this.
- Volunteer: Giving back to your community and feeling a sense of purpose via volunteering. Additionally, it offers the chance to meet new people who share your ideals.
- Stay Active: Take part in group-based physical activities or fitness sessions. Your physical health as well as social engagement are both improved by this.

- Embrace Technology: Keep in contact with family and friends through video calls, social media, or online forums, particularly if distance prevents in-person meetings.
- Seek Professional Help: If you're having trouble with isolation or loneliness, think about talking to a therapist or counselor who can provide support and advice.

Emotional aspects include:

- Practise Self-Compassion: Show yourself compassion and accept your emotions. Self-compassion may help you face the difficulties that come with becoming older while maintaining your resilience.
- Manage Stress: To manage stress and anxiety, use stress-reduction methods such as yoga, deep breathing, meditation, and mindfulness.
- Cultivate Emotional Resilience: Develop coping mechanisms, have a positive mindset, and accept change as a natural

part of life to increase emotional resilience.

- Express Your Emotions: Don't keep your emotions within. It's beneficial to express your feelings, whether it be by journaling, confiding in a close friend, or going to a therapist.
- Set Realistic Expectations: As you become older, modify your expectations. Recognize that alterations in one's physical and mental state are a normal aspect of life.
- Find Meaning and Purpose: Take part in activities that give you a feeling of fulfillment and meaning, whether via your employment, hobbies, volunteer work, or time spent with loved ones.
- Keep Your Mind Active: Keep Your Mind Active** through reading, solving puzzles, picking up new skills, or engaging in creative pursuits. Emotional well-being may be improved through mental stimulation.
- Making time for enjoyable self-care activities, such as taking a bath, going for a walk, or engaging in a favorite activity, should be a priority.

- Stay Open to New Experiences: Even as you become older, be open to attempting new things and pursuing new hobbies. This may keep things interesting and new.
- Seek Professional Help: If you're experiencing emotional difficulties like despair, anxiety, or sorrow, think about seeing a mental health expert. Therapy may provide beneficial guidance and coping mechanisms for emotional wellbeing.

Plateaus and Stalls

When pursuing weight reduction or fitness objectives, especially those connected to intermittent fasting, plateaus, and stalls are frequent occurrences. They may be annoying, but you can get beyond them if you use the appropriate techniques. Here's how to handle stalls and plateaus:

- Evaluate Your Progress First: Examine your present food and exercise routines more carefully. Have you adhered to your fasting schedule and healthy eating plan consistently? Have you lately made any adjustments that might have hindered your advancement?

- Be Patient: Stalls and plateaus are common in any fitness or weight reduction endeavor. Weight reduction is not always linear, and it may take some time for your body to become used to the changes.
- Check Your Calories: You could sometimes require fewer calories when you lose weight. If your objective is to lose weight, reassess your daily caloric intake and ensure that you are still in a calorie deficit. You may need to change the sorts of meals you're eating or your portion sizes.
- Change Up Your Workouts: Change up your fitness program if you're going to do it. Exercise repetitions might cause your body to adapt, resulting in a plateau. To push your muscles, try new things, alter the intensity of your workouts, or include resistance training.
- Keep Tabs on Your Food Intake: To keep track of your diet, keep a food journal. You may use this to find hidden calorie sources or locations where you could be overeating.

- Remain Hydrated: Dehydration may sometimes be confused with hunger. Make sure you're getting enough water each day.
- Take Stress and Sleep into Account: Stress and a lack of sleep might hinder your body's capacity to burn fat. Utilise approaches for reducing stress, and give adequate sleep priority.
- Plateau-Busting Techniques: Experiment with various intermittent fasting strategies, such as adjusting your fasting window.
1. To avoid metabolic adaptation, think about planning periodic "refeed" days when you temporarily boost your calorie intake.
2. Include strength training or high-intensity interval training (HIIT) exercises regularly to increase your metabolism.
- Seek Professional Advice: Consider talking to a licensed dietician or fitness expert if you've experienced a protracted plateau and are having trouble moving forward. They can provide you with personalized guidance and a new point of view.

- Be Consistent and Stay Positive: Keep in mind that plateaus are a normal part of the trip and don't indicate failure. Have your eyes on the prize and have an optimistic outlook.
- Set Non-Scale Objectives: Redirect your attention away from the scale and toward fitness-related non-scale objectives, such as greater strength, endurance, or flexibility. The satisfaction of achieving these objectives may be inspiring.
- Celebrate Little Wins: Celebrate and acknowledge the advancements you have already achieved. Even if the scale isn't moving as much as you'd want it to, it's important to acknowledge and appreciate your efforts.

Chapter 8

Combining Intermittent Fasting with Exercise

In terms of promoting fat loss, reducing insulin resistance, and boosting growth hormones, combining intermittent fasting with exercise has several advantages. Benefits may be further increased by choosing the correct meals both during fasting and when eating.

What you eat in your mouth or don't put in your mouth is not the only factor in weight loss. Consistent exercise is essential to long-term weight control success, regardless of your level of fitness or experience with exercise.

Many individuals like getting up in the morning and starting their day with a run, a trip to the gym, or the use of a fitness video. What to do about exercise is a real worry for women beginning intermittent fasting. It has long been advised against exercising on an empty stomach.

Women who follow the typical diet (3 meals a day with snacks in between) often describe feeling dizzy or queasy when they increase their heart rate on an empty stomach. However, the same things are not experienced by women who follow an intermittent fasting diet. Individuals eventually start to feel energized and have more endurance and stamina.

The Role of Exercise in Your Health

Here are some incredible advantages of exercising when fasting.

- You Burn More Studies indicate that exercising when fasting may increase fat loss by up to 20%. To have the same benefits, you would need to exercise substantially more.
- You Reduce Insulin Resistance: Diabetes and other metabolic diseases are caused by insulin resistance. Having a waistline larger than 35 inches may indicate insulin resistance in women. Intermittent fasting may lower insulin resistance, according to studies.
- You Don't Gain Weight When You Indulge-Many individuals discover that they may enjoy their favorite foods or second helpings guilt-free within their eating window.

- You Initiate the Human Growth Hormone (HGH) Release. This hormone's release increases fat burning and has anti-aging effects.

Choosing the Best Exercise Routine

While exercising while on an intermittent fast may increase fat loss, it's also conceivable that you won't be able to work out as hard due to a lack of energy. To succeed, pay attention to your body.

- Aerobic: This kind of exercise uses your muscles' oxygen supply to power your movements, such as running, cycling, swimming, or dancing. Enhancing cardiovascular health, endurance, and calorie burning via aerobic exercise.
- Anaerobic: During anaerobic activity, your muscles primarily use glucose as fuel. It helps increase muscular strength, power, and calorie burning and includes exercises like running, weightlifting, or leaping.
- Strength: Strength workouts, such as weightlifting, bodyweight exercises, or

utilizing resistance bands, include resistance to test your muscles. They support metabolism, bone density, and muscular development.

- Flexibility: Activities like yoga, pilates, or tai chi concentrate on stretching your muscles and joints. They enhance your posture, and range of motion, and assist in avoiding accidents.
- Balance: Balance exercises, such as utilizing stability balls or balance boards, are meant to preserve stability and coordination. They improve response time, agility, and core strength.

You may burn calories, gain muscle, improve cardiovascular health, elevate mood, and boost cognitive function by exercising. Similar to IF, exercise has advantages such as weight reduction, greater cellular repair, hormone balance, and improved cognitive function.

Performing Exercise Safely for Women Over 50

For women over 50 to maintain their health, fitness, and general well-being, safe exercise is crucial. The following advice will help you exercise safely at this period of your life:

- Consult a Healthcare Professional: Before beginning any fitness program, particularly if you have underlying medical concerns or haven't been active recently, speak with your healthcare practitioner. They can advise you on appropriate workouts and any safety measures you should take.
- Select Appropriate Activities: Pick workouts that suit your degree of fitness, your hobbies, and your physical capabilities. Think about exercises like low-impact aerobics, yoga, Pilates, swimming, cycling, and walking.
- Warm-Up and Cool-Down: Start each workout session with an appropriate warm-up to improve blood flow to your muscles and joints. Stretching is used in the cool-down phase to increase flexibility and lessen discomfort in the muscles.

- **Strength Training:** Include strength training activities in your regimen to keep your metabolism, bone density, and muscular mass in good shape. As your strength improves, start with little weights or resistance bands and progressively increase.
- **Core and Balance Training:** To increase stability and lower the danger of falling, concentrate on core and balance exercises. This is crucial for elderly persons in particular.
- **Listen to Your Body:** While exercising, pay close attention to how your body is feeling. Stop right away and get medical help if required if you feel any unexpected symptoms, such as pain, dizziness, shortness of breath, or any other discomfort.
- **Keep Hydrated:** To keep properly hydrated, particularly in warmer weather, drink water before, during, and after exercise.
- **Good Form:** To avoid injury, learn and put into practice good workout form. If you're hesitant, think about consulting a certified fitness expert who can advise you.

- Progress Gradually: Prevent overexertion and injury by increasing the length, frequency, and intensity of your exercises. Aim for sustained, steady growth.
- Include Flexibility Work: Stretching exercises may increase the range of motion and lower injury risk. Static stretches should be done after your exercises.
- Footwear and Clothes: Dress in breathable, supportive footwear and clothes that are appropriate for the activity you have selected.
- Balance Safety: For exercises like resistance training or cycling, use the correct safety gear and measures. If you're lifting big objects, think about utilizing a spotter.
- Pacing: Go at your own pace when working out. Don't push yourself too hard too soon; instead, give yourself time to recuperate if necessary.
- Drugs: If you take any drugs, be aware of any possible adverse effects that can affect your ability to exercise safely or effectively. If you have any concerns about exercising, speak with your healthcare professional.

- Regular Check-Ups: Arrange frequent visits with your doctor to assess your general health and go through any modifications you've made to your fitness regimen.
- Enjoyment and Variety: To make exercise a lasting part of your lifestyle, choose activities you love. To combat boredom and keep exercises interesting, add diversity.
- Social Engagement: To increase motivation and social connection, think about joining programs or clubs that focus on physical activity.

Chapter 9

Maintaining Long-Term Success

For women over 50 in particular, maintaining long-term success in health and fitness requires establishing sustainable habits and making adjustments to your way of life that you can maintain over time. Here are some tips to aid in your long-term success and maintenance:

- Set Pratical Goals: Make sure your objectives are attainable, precise, and practical and are based on your needs and talents. To keep track of your progress, divide your objectives into more achievable, smaller milestones.
- Consistency is Key: Long-term success requires consistency. Make good food and exercise a regular part of your lifestyle rather than a one-time effort.
- Mindful Eating: Pay attention to what and how you eat when you practice mindful eating. Avoid emotional or thoughtless eating by tuning into your body's hunger and fullness signals.
- Portion Control: Watch the size of your portions to prevent overeating. If doing so

enables you to properly control portion sizes, use smaller plates and utensils.

- Keep a Food Journal: Monitoring your dietary consumption will help you maintain accountability and see areas where you might need to make changes.
- Stay Hydrated: Consume sufficient amounts of water throughout the day to promote general health and avoid dehydration, which may sometimes be confused with hunger.
- Balance Macronutrients: Make sure your meals include a good mix of complex carbs, lean proteins, and heart-healthy fats to provide you with long-lasting energy and enjoyment.
- Prioritize Sleep: To promote hormone balance, energy levels, and general well-being, prioritize getting enough quality sleep.
- Manage Stress: Use stress-reduction methods like yoga, meditation, or deep breathing exercises to lessen the negative effects of stress on your health.
- Celebrate Non-Scale Victories: Don't only concentrate on your weight. Celebrate accomplishments that don't relate to

weight loss, such as greater strength, improved mood, or more vitality.

- Incorporate Strength Training: Strength training keeps muscular mass, which may deteriorate as we age, in check. As part of your program, do resistance workouts to enhance your metabolism and functional fitness.
- Regular Check-Ups: Make appointments with your doctor for routine check-ups to monitor your general health, including your blood pressure, cholesterol, and other critical indicators.
- Stay Informed: Stay current on the most recent findings and advice about women's health, diet, and exercise.
- Adapt to Changing Requirments: Be adaptable and ready to tweak your workout and dietary regimen as your requirements alter as you get older.
- Social Support: Participate in a support group or interact with people who have similar fitness and health objectives. Social support may help with accountability and motivation.
- Recognise that setbacks are a necessary part of the process. Do not lose heart if you fail or encounter difficulties. Take

what you've learned from them and keep going.

- Seek Professional Guidance: If necessary, see a licensed therapist, certified personal trainer, or a registered dietician who focuses on the health and aging of women. They can provide tailored help and direction.
- Make health and fitness a fun part of your life by enjoying the journey. Find things you like doing, enjoy eating properly and welcome the path to long-term wellness.

Being Consistent and Flexible

Long-term success in many areas of life, including health and fitness, depends on being both consistent and adaptable. These two characteristics may support one another and aid you in overcoming obstacles and adjusting to changes in your life. The following describes how to find a balance between rigidity and adaptability:

Consistency:

- Establish a regimen: Establish a regimen that incorporates your exercise and health objectives. Your daily or weekly plan should be consistent if you want to develop good habits.

- Set Specific Objectives: Establish definite, attainable objectives for yourself. These objectives may guide you and keep you on course.
- Prioritize Your Priorities: List your primary concerns, such as your health and exercise. You're more likely to work consistently towards a goal when it's a priority. Find methods to hold yourself responsible, whether it's through keeping track of your progress, utilizing a fitness app, or teaming up with a workout partner.
- Practice Discipline:: Consistency is greatly aided by discipline. There may be times when you lack motivation, but discipline will enable you to continue with your program.
- Celebrate Small Wins: Recognise and enjoy your successes, regardless of how modest they may appear. You could be inspired to maintain consistency by this encouraging feedback.
- Create Habits: Habit formation often leads to consistency. Actions may become

automatic behaviors with repetition, which require less effort.

Flexibility:

- Adapt to Change: Because life is dynamic, things may alter. Allow yourself to change your plans as required without becoming discouraged.
- Manage Setbacks: Recognise that setbacks will occur and use them as a chance to improve. Don't allow one obstacle to cause your whole trip to fail.
- Listen to Your Body: Pay attention to the cues coming from your body. It's OK to change your plans or take a break if you're feeling worn out, hurt, or ill.
- Explore Alternatives: If your existing strategy isn't functioning or doesn't fit your lifestyle anymore, be open to investigating substitute practices.
- Prioritize activities that you love and that are in line with your objectives. It's more difficult to maintain consistency when you don't love something.
- Practise Mindfulness: Develop mindfulness to maintain present-moment

awareness and make quick decisions in the face of changing situations.

- Be Patient and Realistic: Recognise that progression may not always be linear and that there may be times when it moves more slowly. Don't be too hard on yourself.

Maintaining Balance

- Flexibility and consistency are not antagonistic forces. In reality, they are capable of cooperating peacefully. Flexibility enables you to adjust to life's volatility, while consistency gives your ambitions structure and a basis.
- Discover a balance that suits your needs. Your personality and situation will determine how flexible and consistent you are.
- Be aware that being overly flexible could impede growth while being too strict might result in burnout. To maintain your commitment to your objectives while being flexible when necessary, try to find a middle ground.

Tracking Your Progress

Whether your objectives are focused on your profession, personal growth, fitness, or health, tracking your progress is a crucial part of attaining and sustaining them. Tracking offers insightful information, inspiration, and accountability. Here's how to efficiently monitor your development:

- Establish Specific, Measurable Goals: Create objectives that are precise, quantifiable, and unambiguous to start. Your objectives should be measurable so you can assess your development honestly. stating "I want to get healthier," for instance, is not as specific as stating "I want to lose 10 pounds in three months."
- Select the Correct Metrics: Determine the most important metrics or indications that are pertinent to your objectives. Your progress should be immediately measured by these measures. Metrics may include weight, physical measurements, exercise performance, money savings, or professional accomplishments, depending on your objectives.

- Establish a tracking system: Choose a method for assessing your development. You may use a variety of techniques, such as:

1. Digital tools and applications: There are several internet resources and apps for keeping track of money, physical activity, and other things. Examples include habit-tracking, budgeting, and fitness applications.

2. Pencil and paper To manually track your progress, keep a notebook, diary, or spreadsheet. This is particularly helpful for measuring growth or reflection in oneself.

3. Visual aids: To help you visualize your path, think about utilizing visual tools like progress charts, vision boards, or calendars.

- Establish Milestones: Divide your long-term objectives into more manageable, shorter milestones. A feeling of success and gradual tracking of progress are both provided by milestones.

- Regularly Update and Review: Develop a routine of updating your tracking system regularly. Plan specified days or times to evaluate your progress. Depending on the aim, this could happen daily, weekly, or monthly.

- Analyse and Make Adjustments: Analyse the data to find patterns and trends while analyzing your progress. Have you reached a plateau or are you making steady progress? Depending on your findings, modify your strategy as necessary.

Honoring Success

Honoring achievement is an essential habit that may improve your self-esteem, drive, and general well-being. Here are some methods to recognize and enjoy your accomplishments:

- Recognise Your Successes: No matter how large or little, take the time to recognize and celebrate your successes. The first step in celebrating your achievement is acknowledgment.

- Celebrate Milestones: Break down your bigger objectives into more manageable milestones, and then recognize each one when it is reached. These occasions may inspire people and give them a feeling of accomplishment.
- Reflect on Your Journey: Think back on the steps you took to get where you are now. Think back on the difficulties you overcame, the lessons you learned, and the development you went through.
- Express Gratitude: Show your appreciation for the chances and assistance that led to your success. Thanking your friends, family, mentors, or coworkers may be a meaningful way to celebrate your accomplishments.
- Share Your Achievements: Don't be afraid to brag about your achievements, particularly if they have helped you along the way. Sharing may motivate others and have a good knock-on impact.
- Reward Yourself: When you reach a key milestone, treat yourself to a well-deserved treat or indulgence. It may be a

great lunch, a day at the spa, or anything else you've been craving.

- Create a Memory: Commemorate your accomplishments with a special moment. It may be a special excursion, a day trip, or a get-together with close friends and family to commemorate your achievement.
- Journal Your Success: List your accomplishments and the emotions you experienced while working towards them. This may act as a reminder of your accomplishments and a motivating factor when things go tough.
- Set New Goals: Build on your achievements while establishing new objectives. Taking pride in your accomplishments helps keep you inspired and enthusiastic about what is ahead.
- Stay Humble: While it's vital to acknowledge and appreciate your accomplishments, keep in mind to maintain your humility and be receptive to further development and learning.
- Give back by using your achievement to assist others. Mentor, encourage, or invigorate someone pursuing like objectives.

- Self-Compassion: Use self-compassion by treating yourself well and accepting that failures and setbacks are inevitable parts of the path. You should be nice to yourself just as you would a friend.

- Maintain a Success Diary: Keep a diary where you routinely record your accomplishments, no matter how little. Reviewing this notebook may increase your drive and sense of self-worth.

- Visual Reminders: Make visual representations of your accomplishments. This might be a success-related piece of art, a trophy, or a vision board.

- Embrace the Process: Honour not just the accomplishment of your objectives, but also the effort it took to get there. Finding happiness and fulfillment in the trip is a significant approach to appreciating your efforts.

- Stay Positive: Keep a positive outlook and draw strength from your accomplishments. You may keep working towards your objectives by adopting a positive outlook.

Chapter 10

Real-Life Success Stories

How One Lady Shed 90 Poinds via Exercise and IF

Gina Buck decided to prioritize herself after she retired. Eight months later, she has so much vitality that her grandkids are unable to keep up with her.

Gina Buck, 63, thought it was time to look after herself as she neared retirement. She has five grandkids and two children. "I make an effort to maintain my health for the sake of both my family and myself. I want to be able to use my energy to interact with them. I want to be able to do everything that everyone else can do when we go camping, she remarked.

Since she was in her 20s, Buck has battled with her weight. She had considerable stress in her role as a working single mother. She also tried a variety of diets, like many other individuals, but none helped her lose weight permanently.

She had never weighed more than 287 pounds, and she was determined to stay under 300. She is at 195 pounds and wants to reach 180. "I feel so much better now that I've lost the additional weight. I haven't been this little in twenty years. I still have more weight to lose, but I love the new me, so I want to keep walking every day to keep the weight off. "I can do a lot more with my grandchildren now that I'm stronger," she said. Now I'm exhausted!"

She said that as a result of losing weight, she now:

- Sleeps better
- Has less back discomfort
- Can shop for clothing in normal places
- Feels at ease donning shorts and a bathing suit

"In the past, I never wore shorts. I wore capris so I wouldn't expose my flabby legs. I also never would have appeared in public wearing a swimming suit. I now feel at ease in my skin after losing 90 pounds. Going outside and being carefree feels nice, she added.

Here's how she went about it.

Buck saw her doctor in August 2021 and requested medicines to start her weight-loss procedure. According to Buck, the medicine increased her energy and reduced her appetite. She also attempted a program with vitamins, a protein smoothie, and a skin patch with weight-loss-promoting chemicals.

Her first 20 pounds of weight loss came from the combo. I simply needed to start again, she said. She still consumes protein smoothies and vitamins, but she has stopped taking her prescription and taking off the patch.

She intensified her regular strolls.

She found it challenging to walk more than 6,000 steps every day while Buck was at work. "I decided that after I retired, I would focus on myself since I would have unlimited time. She remarked, "I can go for a stroll all day.

She committed to walking 10,000 steps every day when she retired in January 2022, and she kept her word. She wakes up early and heads outside for a stroll as soon as it's light enough to view the ocean since she lives close to Myrtle Ocean, South Carolina. "My kids make fun of me. They claim that Mom won't give up until she completes her steps. But I could stroll down the sand for hours," she said.

When she realized she was walking more than 15,000 steps per day by August, she decided to make it her new objective. After that, everything is a bonus. I take 30,000 steps on certain days, she said.

She works out at Planet Fitness twice a week for approximately an hour and a half, lifting weights to strengthen her arms, legs, stomach, and tummy. Additionally, she bowls twice a week throughout the autumn and winter.

Carolann

I just recently learned that the method I've always eaten has a name: "intermittent fasting." I just refer to it as eating. I've never been a breakfast person because I've never been a morning person. Both my mental and bodily hunger are absent in the morning. Around midday, I first feel the need to eat and am conscious of my appetite. Between noon and one o'clock, I eat my breakfast—cereal, fruit, and milk—as my lunch.

I normally have yogurt at about 3 or 4 p.m., along with some dried fruit (usually figs or prunes), and if I'm still hungry, maybe a tiny handful of almonds or peanuts.

I have supper at roughly 7:00 p.m. Typically, I eat anything I want in a healthy portion size with a mix of protein, carbohydrates, and vegetables. I often prepare extra food and freeze it for later use.

I had a little, thin steak with some potatoes and a salad today as an example of a meal. Preparation took roughly 10 minutes. I ate a large bowl of chicken noodle soup with a salad last night. I had cooked a large quantity of the soup last week and frozen the leftovers in portions. I may have chicken meatballs and rigatoni for dinner tomorrow (store-bought, but of a healthy brand with no strange additives). For supper, I also like eating cheese omelets or bean and cheese tostadas with some avocado.

Planning a tonne of nutritious meals can help you have enough food on hand for the next week. It implies that there is less temptation to just consume quick food, pricey, calorie-dense takeaway, or dine out when you are hungry and weary. All those activities are detrimental to your diet if they become a regular part of your routine.

Only about once a week do I eat out. That has a significant impact. I used to eat out often, and this caused my weight to gradually increase. You may have fun while saving money by cooking.

After supper, if I have a demanding sweet tooth, I'll often have something no later than 7 or 8 p.m. I have some fruit (a juicy orange, an apple, or any delicious summer fruit like peaches or cherries, if they are in season) to satisfy the need. I often indulge in something sweet on the weekends, such as ice cream, cookies, or chocolate candies in moderation rather than going on a full-blown binge.

I don't drink, therefore I don't need to set aside calories for booze. I'm content to spend those calories on indulgent cuisine instead.

That's basically how my unintended intermittent fast has gone. I normally finish my whole meal between noon and eight o'clock. I am now in my fifties and have never been overweight.

If I had been a breakfast person, would the results have been the same? I have no way of knowing, but I do notice that on days when I have to have breakfast early in the morning (for example, if I'm traveling and need to fill up before a busy or taxing day), I start to feel hungry about midday for lunch. I'm certain that if I began "waking up" my digestive system in the morning, I would eat more calories.

Hope this was helpful. I wish you well with your new eating plan!

Inspiring Narratives from Women Over 50 on How They Attained Ageless Vitality

Although particular accounts of women over 50 gaining ageless vigor with intermittent fasting may not be well-documented, the idea of adopting intermittent fasting as a tool for health and vitality is becoming more and more popular among older people. Here is a broad story that summarises the circumstances faced by many women in this age range:

- **Intermittent fasting: Samantha's Path to Ageless Vitality**

Although 52-year-old Samantha had always been mindful of her health, as she approached middle age, she felt the need for a change. She had heard about intermittent fasting and wanted to try it out to maintain youthfulness throughout her whole life. She started on her adventure with a 16/8 intermittent fasting program, which included a 16-hour fast followed by an 8-hour window for eating. Since this schedule permitted her to forego breakfast and have her first meal at noon, she found it very simple to adjust to it.

Samantha concentrated on eating nutrient-dense meals throughout her eating window. She included a lot of fresh produce, lean meats, and good fats in her meals. She started to make portion management a major part of her eating routine. She coupled regular exercise with intermittent fasting. She combined strength training exercises with aerobic workouts like brisk walking to preserve her bone density and muscle mass. She understood how crucial it was to control stress and have a good outlook. She participated in hobbies she enjoyed, including reading and spending time with loved ones, as well as mindfulness meditation. By keeping a log of her eating, exercising, and fasting schedules, Samantha was able to monitor her progress. To track changes in her body composition, she also periodically took measurements.

Samantha noted considerable increases in her energy levels, mental clarity, and general well-being for many months. She shed the extra pounds, and her skin looked more glowing. Improvements in her health indicators, such as blood pressure and cholesterol levels, were found at her yearly physical. Samantha's story encouraged her loved ones to experiment with intermittent fasting and lead better lives. She became an ambassador in her community for active aging and healthy aging.

The experiences of many women over 50 who have adopted intermittent fasting as part of their search for ageless vigor are reflected in Samantha's tale. The concepts of intermittent fasting, when paired with a balanced diet, regular exercise, and mental well-being, may enhance health and energy in later life, however, individual outcomes may vary.

No matter your age or gender, intermittent fasting has become more and more popular as a way of living that may enhance your health and energy. Following are some motivational testimonies from women over 50 who have adopted intermittent fasting and discovered youthful vigor as a result:

- **Susan at 57 and Her Transformation**

For most of her life, Susan, a 57-year-old lady, has battled with her weight. She felt as if her metabolism had slowed down after entering menopause, and she was beginning to lose hope. She did, however, learn about intermittent fasting and decided to give it a go. She adhered to a 16:8 fasting schedule for a whole year while still maintaining a healthy diet and consistent exercise.

Along with losing extra weight, Susan also experienced a surge in energy, mental clarity, and self-confidence. She now promotes intermittent fasting as a means of good aging.

- **Maria's Path to Well-Being at 60**

At the age of 60, Maria was experiencing some health problems, including high blood pressure and joint discomfort. She started a 14:10 fasting schedule that gave her a 10-hour window in which to eat since she was determined to enhance her health.

Maria concentrated on eating meals that were high in nutrients, such as veggies, lean meats, and healthy fats. Her joint pain considerably decreased, her blood pressure stabilized, and her energy levels increased within a year. Many elderly ladies who want to regain their vigor via intermittent fasting find encouragement in Maria's narrative.

- **Karen's Active Retirement at Age 68**

At the age of 68, Karen retired and decided to enjoy her newfound independence. She began experimenting with various intermittent fasting regimens, such as the 5:2 diet, in which she had regular meals for five days and calorie-restricted meals on two separate occasions. Karen discovered that IF enhanced her emotions and cognitive performance in addition to helping her maintain a healthy weight. She now travels, picks up new talents, and lives life to the fullest throughout her retirement.

4. Linda's 55-year fitness journey

Fitness fanatic Linda, 55, added intermittent fasting to her regimen to improve her athletic performance. She adhered to a 20:4 fasting regimen that gave her a 4-hour window each day during which she could eat. Linda discovered that going without food improved her endurance, decreased inflammation, and helped her keep her muscular mass. She keeps taking part in triathlons and marathons, demonstrating that there is no upper age limit for keeping healthy and active.

- **Patricia's Mental Acuity at the Age of 63**

Patricia, who was 63 years old, had memory loss and brain fog. She started intermittent fasting with a concentration on brain-boosting foods like blueberries, fatty salmon, and almonds out of concern about cognitive deterioration. When Patricia followed a 16:8 fasting schedule, her memory and mental clarity significantly improved. Her experience demonstrates the potential advantages of intermittent fasting for cognition, even for those in their 60s and beyond.

These testimonies from women over 50 show that intermittent fasting may be an effective method for maintaining youthful vigor no matter your age. Before beginning any fasting program, particularly if you have underlying health issues, you must speak with a healthcare provider. However, many women discover that intermittent fasting may help them preserve their energy and general well-being as they age when combined with commitment, a healthy diet, and consistent exercise.

Frequently Asked Question

- **How long should women over 50 observe a fast?**

The ideal length of a fast for women over 50 is not a fixed number of hours. Everything depends on your demands and objectives. What are you attempting to achieve, and what can you stick to? Start small, do some research, and gauge your reaction.

- **Does intermittent fasting benefit menopausal women?**

According to recent studies, intermittent fasting may be beneficial for menopausal women.[6] It has been demonstrated to lessen the chance of developing chronic illnesses that menopausal women often experience as well as fight against the symptoms of several metabolic and hormonal changes.

- **Using intermittent fasting, can women over 50 lose weight?**

Without a doubt, intermittent fasting may help women over 50 lose weight.[9] In general, intermittent fasting lowers total calorie consumption, boosts fat burning, and assists in maintaining muscle mass.

- **Which intermittent fasting pattern is most beneficial during menopause?**

16:8 The most practical approach for menopausal women is thought to be intermittent fasting since it is much easier to stick to.

- **How should a lady in her fifties do intermittent fasting?**

It's entirely up to her how to practice intermittent fasting at age 50! We advise beginning with shorter fasts, paying attention to your body, and making sure to consume a lot of healthy meals that are high in nutrients.

- **Should Older Women Fast at the Same Times as Younger Adults?**

Individual demands and tastes may be accommodated by modifying fasting patterns. While some women over 50 may prefer shorter fasting windows, such as 14/10 or 12/12, others may find that longer fasting windows, such as 16/8, are more beneficial to them.

- **What Should I Eat During the Eating Window?**

During your eating window, concentrate on nutrient-dense meals. To help with general health and nutritional requirements, include a lot of fruits, vegetables, lean meats, whole grains, and healthy fats in your meals.

- **Can Intermittent Fasting Aid in Weight Management Following Menopause?**

Particularly during and after menopause, when hormonal changes might impact metabolism, intermittent fasting can be a helpful technique for weight control in women over 50. But for long-term weight control, it's essential to continue eating a balanced diet and going out often in addition to fasting.

- **How Can I Prevent Muscle Loss During Intermittent Fasting?**

Prioritise strength training workouts within your eating window to reduce muscle loss. Make sure you get enough protein to assist muscle development and maintenance.

- **Can Intermittent Fasting Aid in Hormone Regulation?**

According to some studies, intermittent fasting may improve insulin sensitivity and hormone balance, which may be especially advantageous for women over 50. Individual reactions, however, might differ.

- **Is It Common for My Hunger Patterns to Change as I Get Older?**

Yes, it is typical for hunger habits to alter as we become older. As they age, some women could discover that they require fewer calories or have less morning hunger. These modifications may be made to intermittent fasting.

- **Should I Take Supplements During Intermittent Fasting?**

The necessity for vitamins might differ from person to person. Whether you are fasting, it is best to speak with a trained dietitian or healthcare professional to find out whether you have any particular nutritional deficits that call for supplementation.

- **Can Intermittent Fasting Increase Insulin Sensitivity?**

It is especially important for women over 50 who may be more susceptible to insulin resistance and type 2 diabetes to consider intermittent fasting's potential to increase insulin sensitivity. Individual reactions, however, could vary.

Accepting Ageless Vitality Through Intermittent Fasting

It's time to savor the richness of your accomplishments and embrace the timeless energy you've developed as we draw the closing curtain on our adventure together. You've started an inspirational path to become a better, more vibrant version of yourself, and it's one to be proud of.

The amazing realm of intermittent fasting, designed especially for the outstanding ladies over 50, has been thoroughly examined throughout this book. You've studied the underlying research, found the numerous methods, and learned how to choose the one that works best for you. You've evaluated your health, made powerful objectives, and taken the first steps towards regaining your feeling of well-being.

Consider the transforming steps you've done along the road when you look back on your trip and keep in mind that success isn't just about arriving at your objective. It's about the fresh energy you've found, the courage you've developed, and the assurance that springs from your enduring vitality.

However, this is only a fresh start; it's not the end. Your experience with IF is continual; it's a constantly changing tango with healthiness. Keep these guidelines in mind as you go forward:

- Maintaining your chosen intermittent fasting practice regularly is important. Success is bred by consistency, and little, lasting adjustments add up to big effects.
- Pay Attention to Your Body: Your body is a sage and a teacher. Pay attention to its

cues and modify your fasting strategy as necessary. You may count on self-care and self-awareness as your guides on this path.

- Seek Assistance: Lean on your network of friends, family, and online groups for support. Discuss your difficulties, celebrate your successes, and gain courage from your peers' accumulated knowledge.
- Adapt to Change: Your objectives and situation could change over time. Be willing to change your fasting plan as necessary to accommodate changing requirements and goals.
- Accept Ageless Vitality: Always keep in mind that age is only a number. Being at your finest all the time is what ageless vitality is all about. Take pride in it and keep taking care of your well-being.

Age brings knowledge, and insight gives you the ability to control your future. Your youthful vigor is proof of your resiliency and inner strength. Continue enjoying it, tending to it, and continuing to live life to the fullest.

May you have energy throughout the day, joy in your heart, and the everlasting spark of ageless vigor in your soul as you continue on your intermittent fasting adventure. The greatest is yet to come in this period that is yours.

Cheers to you and your exciting future chapters! Your continuing tale of youth-defying energy is one worth savoring.

I hope you continue to be successful and happy.

(Aubrey Wheatly)

www.ingramcontent.com/pod-product-compliance
Lightning Source LLC
Chambersburg PA
CBHW070846260726

48661CB00004B/1263